DOPAMINE DETOX GUIDE

A DETAILED GUIDE TO GETTING YOUR BRAIN TO FUNCTION OPTIMALLY BY TAKING OUT DISTRACTIONS AND TAKE FULL CONTROL OF YOUR LIFE

CASTRO ATKIN

Made with ♥ on the Notion Press Platform
www.notionpress.com

Contents

Title Page

DOPAMINE DETOX GUIDE

A detailed guide to getting your brain to function optimally by taking out distractions and take full control of your life

Castro Atkin

CHAPTER ONE

INTRODUCTION TO DOPAMINE DETOX

Are you frustrated with the amount of time you spend on the Internet, yet you find that you can't stop yourself from doing it?

Is it no longer entertaining?

Do you know what you should be doing, but instead you choose to engage in behavior that would provide you with instant gratification?

Do you ever feel like you're missing out on the excitement when you participate in routine activities that other people enjoy?

These are the indications that a dopamine detox is necessary for you.

So what precisely does "dopamine detox" mean?

The original dopamine detox seems to be a decent guideline for healthy digital behaviors; nonetheless, we believe that it will not be enough to re-establish healthy surfing habits and get over an addiction to the internet.

It's nothing more than a clever tagline designed to grab our attention.

On the other hand, there is an appropriate manner to carry it out, and that is the subject of this tutorial.

What to know about Dopamine and its function in the brain

Dopamine is a neurotransmitter, which is a chemical messenger in the brain that helps to carry messages between nerve cells. Neurotransmitters include serotonin, acetylcholine, and vasopressin.

It is involved in a wide variety of brain activities, among of the most important of which include pleasure, pleasure regulation, reward, and motivation.

Dopamine is generated in the brain by neurons with a specific chemical makeup known as dopaminergic neurons.

These neurons are responsible for releasing dopamine into certain parts of the brain, such as the striatum and the prefrontal cortex, where it may then attach to dopamine receptors that are located on other neurons.

Dopamine is a neurotransmitter that is secreted into the bloodstream in response to a rewarding or enjoyable event. It is responsible for producing a feeling of pleasure and for reinforcing the behavior that led to the release of dopamine.

Because of this property, dopamine is often referred to as the "feel-good" molecule.

Nevertheless, prolonged or excessive exposure to dopamine may cause changes in the reward system of the brain. These changes can result in a diminished capacity to perceive pleasure as well as an increased risk of addiction as well as sadness, anxiety, and other mental health issues.

Dopamine detox might be useful in this situation since its primary goals are to minimize the amount of stimulus that the brain is subjected to and to reset the reward system.

Significance of dopamine detox

The potential of dopamine detox to reset the brain's reward system is one of its most important benefits. When the brain is subjected to an excessive amount of stimulation, the reward system might become insensitive to its natural pleasures.

This may lead to an increased risk of addiction as well as depression, anxiety, and other mental health disorders. [Cause and effect]

Dopamine detox may be helpful in reducing the amount of excessive stimulation that the brain is subjected to. This stimulation can originate from a variety of sources, including social media, video games, processed foods, and other addictive drugs or activities.

Dopamine detox may assist to restore the brain's sensitivity to natural pleasures, hence lowering the risk of both addiction and mental health issues. This is accomplished by minimizing or removing the sources of stimulation that cause dopamine release.

Dopamine detox has the potential to enhance one's mental health, as well as their ability to concentrate, their level of productivity, their level of creativity, and their general well-being.

Dopamine detox may assist to increase mental clarity and decrease stress by minimizing the amount of distractions and excessive stimulation in the environment. This can lead to a stronger feeling of peace and equilibrium in day-to-day living.

Dopamine detox is important because it has the ability to reset the reward system in the brain and to boost general mental and physical health. This is the main reason for its relevance.

Overview of the benefits and positive effects of Dopamine detox

Detoxing from dopamine may have a variety of positive effects on one's mental and physical health, including the following:

1. increased mental clarity and concentration Dopamine detox may assist to boost attention and productivity by lowering the number of stimuli and distractions that the brain is exposed to.

2. Decreased levels of stress and anxiety Dopamine detox may assist in lowering levels of tension and anxiety by fostering a stronger feeling of tranquility and equilibrium.

3. Enhanced creativity and productivity dopamine detox may assist in enhancing creativity and productivity by lowering the number of distractions experienced and increasing the level of mental clarity experienced.

4. An improvement in the quality of sleep Dopamine detox may assist to enhance sleep quality and promote improved overall health by limiting exposure to artificial stimuli such as the blue light emitted by electronic devices.

5. Improved self-awareness and the ability to develop mindfulness: Dopamine detox may aid in the cultivation of mindfulness and bring about an increase in self-awareness by encouraging a better feeling of presence and awareness.

Dopamine detox may, in general, contribute to a stronger feeling of well-being and balance in everyday life. Moreover, it may assist to lower the risk of addiction, depression, anxiety, and other mental health disorders.

CHAPTER TWO

What to know about dopamine detox

The term "dopamine detox" refers to a period of time during which a person deliberately limits or removes their exposure to sources of excessive stimulation. Some examples of such sources are social media, video games, processed meals, and other addictive drugs or activities.

The purpose of dopamine detox is to limit the amount of time that the brain is subjected to excessive stimulation and to reset the reward system. The reward system might become insensitive to natural pleasures if it is exposed to stimulation for an extended period of time or in excessive amounts.

This may assist to restore the brain's sensitivity to natural pleasures and lessen the likelihood of addiction as well as other mental health issues such as sadness and anxiety.

Dopamine detoxification may be accomplished in a variety of ways, such as via a digital detox, a food and drink detox, or a detox in the environment, and it can entail a wide variety of activities, such as meditation, physical activity, and time spent outside.

How does dopamine detox function

Dopamine detoxification is effective because it lessens or eliminates the brain's exposure to sources of excessive stimulation. These kinds of stimulation may cause alterations in the brain's reward system and lessen the brain's sensitivity to the joys that come from natural experiences.

The brain produces dopamine, a neurotransmitter that generates a sensation of pleasure and promotes the activity that led to the production of dopamine, when it is subjected to excessive stimulation, such as that which may be obtained through social media, video games, or processed foods, among other sources.

The reward system in the brain has the potential to grow desensitized to the joys that are naturally occurring over time. As a result, more stimulation is required to maintain the same degree of pleasure.

This may lead to an increased risk of addiction as well as depression, anxiety, and other mental health disorders. [Cause and effect]

The purpose of dopamine detox is to minimize the amount of stimulus that the brain is subjected to and to reset the reward system.

Getting rid of these toxins may be accomplished in a variety of ways, including by engaging in a "digital detox," "food and drink detox," or "environmental detox."

For instance, in order to participate in a digital detox, one must limit or refrain from using digital devices such as smartphones, computers, and televisions. In contrast, one must limit or refrain from participating in a food and drink detox in order to limit or refrain from consuming processed foods and caffeine.

During a dopamine detox, people may also participate in activities such as meditation, physical exercise, and spending time in nature. These activities may assist to develop a stronger sense of peace and balance, as well as lessen feelings of tension and worry.

Dopamine detox works by limiting the amount of excessive stimulation that the brain is subjected to. This, in turn, helps to reset the reward system and restores the brain's sensitivity to the joys that come from natural experiences.

This may lead to a stronger feeling of well-being and lessen the risk of addiction, depression, anxiety, and other mental health disorders. [Cause and effect]

CHAPTER THREE

Why engage in a dopamine fast?

Doping yourself up on dopamine may be something you want to try for a few different reasons:

- You can't help yourself and can't stop surfing
- You want to make everyday activities more fascinating and exciting
- You are sick of the way you spend your time
- You can't help yourself and can't stop surfing (and not need to have your phone in your hand constantly just to feel engaged)

There are particular reasons for this, but the overarching goal remains the same: to have a more positive connection with your smartphone, the Internet, and the digital world as a whole.

These are the objectives:

1. To disrupt the habit of obsessive activities such as mindlessly picking up your phone or browsing the web, which may become difficult to quit.

Examples of rabbit holes include videos on YouTube.

2. The realization that the fact that we desire or want something does not guarantee that we will like it once we are actually doing it.

As an example, we can be exaggerating how enjoyable it would be to relive the experience of playing a certain game again.

In point of fact, all of it is merely our sense of nostalgia coming into play.

3. to give the brain time to replenish its supply of dopamine receptors so that everyday activities may once again become more enjoyable.

For example, you decide to pick up an old pastime since you've discovered that you've missed it.

The addiction-free life may be achieved with this simple method:

A desire to change, an understanding of addiction, the ability to break the pattern of compulsive behavior, the construction of a better life, and improved emotional control all contribute to success.

Dopamine detoxification involves acting on the urge to change and breaking the pattern of compulsive behavior that the desire has created.

This provides you with breathing space, allows you to develop a better life, and, if you actively attempt to accomplish these things, teaches you how to better control your emotions.

Doing dopamine detox the right way

How long should you give yourself to detox off dopamine?

In general, 2-12 weeks.

It takes some time for the wiring in our brains to change.

We chose to make our challenge last for 14 days since the least amount of time necessary to see obvious results is two weeks.

30 days is a sufficient amount of time to see changes and is a decent length for a monthly challenge.

We strongly suggest moving in this direction.

The normal treatment for Internet addiction lasts for a period of twelve weeks (which is also close to popular 90 days or 100 days challenges).

There is often ample time to make significant changes in your life, but many individuals find that the commitment required is too overwhelming.

1. Eliminate all of your zombie-inducing behaviors immediately.

A good rule of thumb to keep in mind is the following:

Remove from your life anything that has the potential to turn you into a zombie for the length of the challenge.

Zombie Mode is when you are unable to stop browsing, viewing, or playing for hours on end despite the fact that you are not actually enjoying what you are doing but are unable to do anything of value.

It's when you find yourself spending hours participating in low-quality dopamine activities.

The most typical forms of distraction are as follows: social media; content aggregators (such as YouTube, Reddit, and Hackernews); Twitch; binge-watching on Netflix; video games; porn; combinations of all of the aforementioned; bouncing from one to another.

You are well aware of what it is that you do.

It's possible that you'll catch yourself convincing yourself that you don't have to give up these things because you'll only have to exercise a little more self-control and everything will be OK.

You may want to give it a go.

On the other hand, this is a common justification because: If you were able to control your conduct, you wouldn't be in this predicament in the first place.

However, these activities are often linked to one another, which means that even if YouTube is the primary source of your problem, accessing social networking websites frequently leads you to YouTube.

In addition, when your dopamine receptors are depleted, it is very difficult to manage your behavior, which is one of the reasons why one of the aims of the dopamine detox is to restore your capacity to control your behavior.

Where can I obtain the inspiration to do this?

It's possible that your life is a mess right now.

Or maybe things are going well, but you're not happy and you get the impression that you're squandering a lot of time.

Another possible indicator is if you find it difficult to stop doing anything, such as watching YouTube videos or playing video games.

It may be an indication that you need it in a significant manner.

Having the motivation to improve oneself is of critical significance.

Check out the following arguments against mindless web browsing if you are still undecided about whether or not you should engage in this activity.

We are not going to sugarcoat the fact that adjustment may be challenging and that you may experience discomfort throughout the transition period.

However:

1. You won't be sorry that you did it.

2. It will be lot simpler for you to do than you imagine it would be.

3. You are free to return at any time to the behaviors you had before.

How to abstain from behaviors that are addictive

Get rid of applications on your phone that are a distraction, and block websites that are a distraction on your computer.

When you hear your brain telling you that you really need to watch Twitch in the evening because [insert any arbitrary reason here], remind it that you can come back to it when your dopamine detox is through. Using a handful of severe steps can help you get through this.

What about activities that are necessary but yet cause obsessive behavior (like constantly checking your email, for example)?

Choose when throughout the day you will give yourself permission to do this and for how long you will give yourself permission to do it.

For instance, you will only be permitted to check your email for a period of 15 minutes at 10 a.m. and again at 4 p.m.

(Here's a helpful hint: to do this, you may utilize the Batch Rule function of our plugin.)

You might also begin a dopamine detox counter in order to serve as a constant reminder that you are making an effort to alter your behavior.

Writing down on a piece of paper the number of days, beginning with zero, that you have been adhering to your new routine is a simple and effective way to track your progress.

Participate in activities that are true to life.

When you have removed all potential sources of addiction, the next issue is, "During a dopamine detox, what exactly should you be doing?"

You do not want to do nothing but laze around all day.

But, it is far simpler to run toward something than than away from it.

It is likely that you will relapse if you do not make an effort to create a life that is more enjoyable without the Internet and if you do not make an effort to overcome the underlying reasons that contribute to obsessive use of technology.

You won't be able to break your poor behaviors for very long.

What exactly do we mean when we talk about a life that is more satisfying?

You may, for instance, engage in pursuits the completion of which leaves you feeling upbeat.

Excellent dopamine detox activities:

- Engaging in conversation with others
- Cooking and eating
- Taking walks
- Reading books
- Keeping a journal
- Working out

There is one thing that all of these hobbies have in common, and that is the fact that they move you away from screens.

All of these activities are examples of what we mean when we talk about seeking high-quality leisure.

Be precise about the ways in which you can make better use of your time.

Ask yourself this question: when you do find yourself becoming a little bored, what are some simple things that you could perform?

Drawing?

Journalling?

Reading?

Tidying?

Now is also a great time to try something new and exciting, such as enrolling in a salsa dancing class, beginning the craft of origami, or picking up the flute.

Make an interest that you've had in the past but haven't done anything with active now.

It is helpful if you develop a real physical list of these activities to refer to later.

When you take a look at the physical list that you have posted on your door or refrigerator, it will serve as a constant reminder of productive activities to use your time.

It's possible that performing the activities listed above won't take up the bulk of your spare time. If this is the case, you may want to consider picking up hobbies or pursuits that you abandoned due of the Internet, such as playing an instrument, sketching, or...

- Improve your existing talents
- Look for new interests (can you recall what they were?)
- Spending time outside is encouraged
- Look for a group to join.

You also have the ability to choose your addiction.

There is an infinite number of things that might be enjoyable; thus, you shouldn't give it too much thought and should instead experiment with various options.

Complete the following statement for a good starting point while looking for possibly intriguing hobbies:

"I've never had the time or the chance to _______________, but it's something I've always wanted to do," you say.

Doing a dopamine detox will allow you to have more time on your hands.

3. Limit your consumption to solely long-form material

This is the point at which the debate becomes contentious since traditional "dopamine fasters" believe that the consumption of long-form information constitutes a dopamine-heavy activity.

Yet, we are here for the long term, and if your goal is to complete the program in four to twelve weeks, living like a monk will make it impossible for you to do so.

The vast majority of individuals are unable to maintain a constant job schedule (although what we call work is often subjective).

Many make the futile attempt to make up for the time they waste during their spare time by increasing their level of productivity, but this strategy is not sustainable.

We need time away from work as well as breaks in order to properly recharge our batteries.

But, even if you begin engaging in more thoughtful forms of recreation, you could find that you fatigue easily if you try to do so constantly.

You don't want to engage in things that require no mental effort since they were the behaviors that got you into problems in the first place.

Instead, you should focus on selecting high-quality information that can be enjoyed most when it is taken in more gradually, such as long-form content.

Books and CDs are also excellent options to consider.

It's a lot of fun to get together in person with friends to play board games.

It's quite acceptable to sit through a single film without any interruptions.

It's not productive to watch many episodes of a Netflix series in rapid succession while also browsing on your phone.

It's perfectly OK to spend all your time just listening to music.

Letting it play in the background nonstop is not acceptable.

We went through the key distinctions between viewing Netflix, television, and movies in a theater.

The compulsivity risk associated with long-form material is much reduced.

The difficulty with activities that are highly dopaminergic is as follows:

Dopamine motivates you to engage in behaviors that will result in the greatest release of dopamine.

The following is a list of the components that contribute to the high dopamine content of a behavior:

• The amount of time that the activity stimulates you • The amount of dopamine that is released as a result of the behavior

• The intensity of the stimulation • The novelty of the behavior

While it is difficult to assess this on an individual level, you should be able to approximate it if you give it a moment of your time and some thought.

Medications cause a significant rise in activity and have a very high potential for stimulation.

The stimulus that may be experienced when playing video games is not only intense, but also lasts for an extremely long time.

Porn is really exciting and quite different from anything else out there.

As compared to longer-form material such as a movie, for example, these activities provide stimulation for a longer period of time, but the effect is not as strong.

CHAPTER FOUR

Carrying out dopamine detox in variety of ways

Dopamine detoxification may be accomplished in a variety of methods, including the following:

1. Participating in a digital detox entails minimizing or omitting one's usage of digital gadgets such as mobile phones, personal computers, and TVs.

This may assist to limit exposure to digital stimulation, which can contribute to increased dopamine release in the brain. Digital stimulation includes things like social media, email, and other forms of digital stimulation.

2. Detoxification of food and drink: This comprises lowering or omitting one's intake of processed foods, sugary beverages, and caffeine.

These chemicals have the potential to trigger an increase in the production of dopamine, which in turn has the potential to dull the brain's reward system.

3. Detoxifying one's surroundings entails limiting one's exposure to environmental elements that have the potential to generate an excessive amount of stimulation. Some examples of these factors are loud sounds, bright lights, and clutter.

This may assist to lessen feelings of tension and anxiety, as well as generate a stronger sense of serenity.

4. Engaging in activities that foster a deeper feeling of present and awareness, such as meditation, yoga, or deep breathing

exercises, is an example of a practice that falls under the category of mindfulness. These activities may also assist to alleviate stress and anxiety.

5. Exercise: This includes participating in physical activity, which may help to increase the release of endorphins, which are natural chemicals that provide a sensation of pleasure and decrease stress. 5. Exercise can help to stimulate the release of endorphins, which can help: 5.

6. Spending time in natural habitats, such as parks, woods, or beaches, which may assist to promote relaxation and decrease stress is the sixth tip. This entails spending time in natural surroundings such as parks, forests, or beaches.

In general, a dopamine detox may be accomplished in a number of different ways, and the one that may prove to be the most successful is likely to be determined by the unique requirements and preferences of the person in question.

Before beginning a dopamine detox, it is critical to discuss the process with a qualified medical professional, particularly if you are currently managing any preexisting medical issues or are on any medications.

Digital detox

A detox from digital gadgets, such as cellphones, laptops, and TVs, is also referred to as a "digital detox."

This may assist to limit exposure to digital stimulation, which can contribute to increased dopamine release in the brain. Digital stimulation includes things like social media, email, and other forms of digital stimulation.

Here are some recommendations for undergoing a digital detox:

1. Establish a goal:

Have a concrete objective for your digital detox, such as lowering the total amount of time spent in front of a screen by a certain percentage or abstaining from social media for a predetermined length of time.

2. Develop a strategy: Establish a plan for how you will decrease your digital usage, such as setting specified times of day for

checking email or social media, or turning off alerts on your phone. For example, you might create defined hours for checking email or social media.

3. Look for activities that aren't related to technology: If you want to reduce the amount of time you spend using technology, you should look for activities that aren't related to technology, such as reading a book, going for a walk, or spending time with friends and family.

4. Eliminate sources of temptation: Eliminate any sources of digital temptation from your surroundings, such as switching off your phone during meals or deleting social media applications from your smartphone. This will help you stay on track with your goals.

5. Have patience: It is possible that it may take some time for you to adapt to a digital detox, so have patience with yourself and don't expect results right away.

Overall, participating in a digital detox program may assist in lessening the amount of excessive stimulation that the brain is subjected to and fostering a stronger feeling of serenity and equilibrium.

It is possible that people may have enhanced mental clarity and concentration, higher sleep quality, and lower levels of stress and anxiety if they minimize the amount of time spent using digital gadgets.

Food and drink detox

Reducing or eliminating the intake of certain foods and beverages that are known to induce an increase in the amount of dopamine that is released in the brain is the goal of a food and drink detox.

They include meals that have been processed, beverages with added sugar, and caffeine.

The following are some suggestions for doing a detoxification of food and drink:

1. Determine which foods cause desires: Determine which items, such as sugary snacks or processed meals, cause cravings and may lead to excessive intake. One way to do this is to keep a food

diary.

2. Make advance meal preparations:

Make sure that you are eating healthy and nutrient-dense foods by preparing your meals in advance. Some examples of these foods are fruits, vegetables, whole grains, and lean meats.

3. Stay away from sugary beverages Stay away from sugary drinks like soda, energy drinks, and sports drinks since they might cause an increase in the amount of dopamine that is released in the brain.

4. Consume less caffeine: If you are a habitual caffeine consumer, you should gradually lower the amount of caffeine you drink in order to prevent withdrawal symptoms such as headaches and weariness.

5. Keep yourself hydrated: Consuming a lot of water can assist the body flush out toxins while also keeping you hydrated.

Be patient: It may take some time to adapt to a food and drink detox, so be patient with yourself and don't expect quick results. Be patient with yourself and don't expect to see benefits right away.

Detoxifying the body's diet may, in general, assist to lessen the amount of unnecessary stimulation that the brain is subjected to and foster a stronger feeling of general wellbeing.

A person's energy levels, the quality of their sleep, and the degree of inflammation in their bodies may all improve as a result of an increase in the consumption of foods that are healthy and nutritious.

Environment detox

Reducing one's exposure to environmental variables that might produce excessive stimulation, such as bright lights, loud sounds, and clutter, is one component of an environment detox.

This may assist to lessen feelings of tension and anxiety, as well as generate a stronger sense of serenity.

Here are some suggestions for undertaking an environment detox:

1. Decrease the amount of time spent in front of devices: To limit the amount of exposure to bright lights, reduce the amount of

time spent in front of displays such as computers, cellphones, and TVs.

2. Make use of natural light: In order to maintain your body's normal sleep-wake cycle, you should make an effort to expose yourself to as much natural light as you can, particularly in the morning.

3. Protect Your Ears by Using Earplugs or Noise-Cancelling Headphones Wearing earplugs or noise-canceling headphones may help protect your hearing from loud sounds, particularly in places that are busy or noisy.

4. Eliminate the clutter in your area Get rid of any belongings or clutter that aren't essential in your house or office in order to create an atmosphere that is more calm and well ordered.

5. Provide a peaceful and relaxing atmosphere Make use of colors that are calming as well as natural elements such as wood and plants to create a soothing and relaxing atmosphere.

6. Have patience: As it may take some time to adapt to a detox atmosphere, it is important to have patience with yourself and not to anticipate results right away.

In general, a detoxification of the surroundings may assist to lessen the amount of overstimulation that the brain is subjected to and foster a stronger feeling of peace and equilibrium.

It is possible for people to enjoy enhanced attention and productivity, higher sleep quality, lower stress and anxiety, and better overall health when they cultivate an atmosphere that is tranquil and well structured.

Advantages of Dopamine detoxification

Dopamine detox has the potential to provide a number of advantages, including the following:

1. Improved attention and output may result from limiting one's exposure to an excessive amount of stimuli; this allows for the possibility of increased productivity in persons.

2. Improvements in mental clarity and attention may be seen by people as a result of a decrease in the amount of dopamine spikes in their systems.

3. Decreased levels of stress and anxiety: Individuals may feel decreased levels of stress and anxiety when their exposure to stressful stimuli is decreased.

4. Better sleep quality Those who limit their participation in stimulating activities in the hours leading up to bedtime may find that their sleep is of higher quality and lasts longer.

5. An improvement in mood It is possible that people would have a more consistent and happy mood as a result of a reduction in the frequency of dopamine spikes.

6. Improved self-awareness Individuals may become more self-aware and in touch with their own wants and desires if they take a break from digital gadgets and other types of stimulation, such as exercise and conversation with others.

Dopamine detoxification, in general, may assist to foster a stronger feeling of well-being and balance, and it may eventually lead to improvements in mental and physical health.

CHAPTER FIVE

Detailed instructions to dopamine detox

The following is an outline of the detoxification process for dopamine:

1. Have a plan for your detox. Figure out how long your detox will last and what kinds of activities you will try to avoid or cut down on.

This might include things like social media, streaming services, video games, processed meals, sugary beverages, coffee, and any other things that provide an excessive amount of stimulation.

2. Get your surroundings ready: Before you start your detox, get your environment ready by getting rid of any temptations and making a setting that is serene and relaxing for yourself.

De-cluttering your house or workplace, designing a location specifically for relaxing, and reducing your exposure to stimuli like bright lights and loud sounds are all potential steps in this direction.

3. Have crystal clear objectives: Establish crystal clear objectives for your detox, such as increasing your productivity, decreasing your stress, or enhancing the quality of your sleep.

Put your objectives in writing and make sure you keep coming back to them so you can maintain your motivation.

4. Make a routine: Make a calendar for yourself that includes things that help you relax, such as meditation, yoga, reading, or spending time in nature. This program may be used on a daily or weekly basis.

5. Look for options that are better for you:

Consider participating in physical exercise, sipping herbal tea, or eating whole foods as some of the healthier alternatives to the foods and activities that you are trying to avoid.

6. Engage in self-care activities: As you are going through the process of detoxing, you should put an emphasis on engaging in self-care activities such as getting enough sleep, eating healthily, and practicing mindfulness.

7. Keep in touch with those you care about Even while it's necessary to restrict the amount of time spent on social media and other sources of excessive stimulation, it's just as crucial to keep in touch with the people you care about.

Make plans to participate in low-stimulation activities with your loved ones, including both friends and family.

8. Assess your progress After you have completed your detox program, it is important to review your progress and think about what aspects worked well and what aspects may need some improvement.

Make use of this knowledge to determine which improvements, if any, are essential to make to your way of life moving ahead.

In general, a dopamine detox may be an effective method for improving equilibrium and well-being in a world with an excessive amount of stimulation.

Individuals may experience the advantages of a dopamine detox and create healthy behaviors over time by defining clear objectives for themselves, creating an atmosphere that is supportive of their efforts, and placing a priority on self-care.

Have a proper Plan for your detox process

Included below are some measures that might assist you in arranging a dopamine detox, should you decide to go through with one:

1. Choose how long you want your detox to endure and set a length goal for it.

It may be a single day, a whole weekend, an entire week, or even longer.

The time is determined by your own objectives and the conditions at hand.

2. Determine the activities or substances that cause dopamine levels to surge in your brain. This is the second step in the process.

This might include things like social media, streaming services, video games, processed meals, sugary beverages, coffee, and any other things that provide an excessive amount of stimulation.

3. Make a list of activities: Throughout your detox, you should make a list of activities that you will either not participate in or restrict to a certain extent.

This list can contain the triggers you discovered in step 2, in addition to any activities that you believe might be too stimulating for you.

4. Make a list of things that you can do instead Make a list of activities that you can do instead of detoxing during the time that you are detoxing.

This may include indulging in physical activities such as walking, yoga, or riding; mental activities such as reading books or keeping a diary; or creative pursuits such as drawing, painting, or writing.

5. Establish parameters:

Establish personal limits and make sure those boundaries are clear to the individuals in your life.

Inform them that you will be taking a break from particular hobbies or drugs and ask for their support while you are in this period of transition.

6. Get your surroundings ready: Get your environment ready by getting rid of any temptations and making a location that is tranquil and pleasant for you to be in.

De-cluttering your house or workplace, designing a location specifically for relaxing, and reducing your exposure to stimuli like bright lights and loud sounds are all potential steps in this direction.

7. Establish a calendar: Develop a timetable for yourself that includes the things you will undertake while detoxing. This

schedule may be daily or weekly.

This will assist you in maintaining your progress and avoiding the triggers that you discovered before.

8. Get support: Throughout the detox process, it is helpful to have the assistance of a friend or member of your family.

This individual has the ability to hold you responsible and offer support at the appropriate times when you need it.

Keep in mind that going through a dopamine detox is a personal experience, and the methods that work for one person may not work for another.

Throughout the detox process, it is important to be nice to yourself and to pay attention to what your body requires.

It is possible that you will discover that you have more energy, that you feel more focused, and that you have a greater feeling of well-being if you take a vacation from excessive stimulation.

Establish unmistakable goals and objectives

A crucial component of a dopamine detox is the establishment of distinct objectives.

The following are some methods that can assist you in establishing your goals:

1. Determine your priorities:

Consider what is most essential to you to get the conversation started.

Which aspects of your life do you feel might need some work?

Your priorities and your objectives need to be in agreement with one another.

2. Be specific:

Be sure that your objectives can be measured and that they are explicit.

For instance, rather of making a goal as general as "decrease stress," make it as precise as "practice meditation for ten minutes every day." This will help you achieve your objective of reducing stress.

3. write them on paper:

Put your objectives in writing and display them in an area where you will be able to view them on a frequent basis.

This will assist you in maintaining your motivation and keeping your concentration.

4. Deconstruct them as follows:

Your ambitions should be broken down into smaller, more attainable stages.

Keeping to your original plan and avoiding a sensation of being overwhelmed will be easier with this assistance.

5. Make sure they are achievable: Ensure that your objectives are reasonable and that you can meet them.

Establishing objectives that are impossible to achieve or too challenging might result in feelings of anger and disappointment.

6. Evaluate and modify: On a regular basis, evaluate your progress toward your objectives, and modify them as need.

As you go forward with your detoxification process, you may discover that your objectives need modification in light of your experiences and overall development.

Keep in mind that the objectives you choose for your dopamine detox are specific to your needs and preferences.

They should be intended to assist you attain a healthy balance in your life and should be linked with the priorities you have set for yourself.

Throughout your detox, you will have more motivation and concentration if you have clearly defined objectives to work toward, which will boost your chances of being successful.

Prepare a schedule

Developing a routine is an essential step in the dopamine detoxification process.

The following are some of the stages that can assist you in developing your schedule:

1. Determine your priorities:

To get started, you should think about the activities that are most important to you.

They have to be the kinds of activities that fit in well with the objectives you have set for the dopamine detox.

2. Establish a timetable: Determine how long your dopamine detox will continue and then establish a timetable for your daily activities.

This may be a day, a weekend, a week, or even longer, depending on the specifics of your situation and the objectives that you have set for yourself.

3. Establish a routine for each day:

Create a timetable for each day of your detox and break it down into daily chunks to make it more manageable.

Make sure that you schedule time in your schedule for things that are essential to you, such as getting exercise, practicing meditation, or hanging out with the people you care about.

4. Keep your expectations in check: double check that your timetable is both reasonable and doable.

If you make the mistake of trying to pack too much into one day, you run the risk of being disheartened and overwhelmed.

5. Add alternative activities: Make sure that your calendar includes alternative activities that will assist you in avoiding the triggers that you identified earlier. These activities may be found in the previous step.

If you're trying to stay away from social media, for instance, you might make time in your calendar to read a book or go on a walk instead.

6. Be flexible: Keep in mind that your agenda is a guide, not a rigid set of rules, and use it as such.

Maintain your flexibility and be open to make changes to your routine if they become required.

7. Commit to following your timetable: After you have developed your plan, you should resolve to follow it as closely as you possibly can.

Throughout the dopamine withdrawal process, this will help you maintain your attention and keep you motivated.

Keep in mind that the plan you've created for yourself is intended to assist you in achieving your objectives and establishing a more healthy balance in your life.

You will have a better chance of succeeding in your dopamine detox and feeling the advantages of lowering the amount of stimulation you are exposed to if you stick to a plan.

Discover options that are healthy and helpful

During your dopamine detox, it might be helpful to find healthy alternatives to the behaviors or routines that you are attempting to break. This can assist you in remaining on track and achieving your objectives.

The following are some measures that can assist you in locating options that are healthier:

1. Make a list of the behaviors or routines you want to avoid: To begin, make a list of the behaviors or routines that you want to avoid while you are going through the dopamine detox process.

This can be anything like social media, junk food, or other things that you find to be too stimulating for you.

2. Do research on healthy alternatives After you have determined the behaviors or routines that you want to eliminate from your life, the next step is to conduct study on healthy alternatives that may take their place.

For instance, if you wish to stay away from social media, you may take up a new pastime instead, such as painting, gardening, or doing yoga.

3. Pick activities you enjoy:

Choose out options that are good for you, that you like, and that are in line with your objectives.

This will make it much simpler for you to adhere to them and avoid engaging in the behaviors or routines that you are attempting to break.

4. Make your preparations in advance:

Be ready in advance for the alternative activities you've selected by gathering the supplies you'll need or arranging the space where you'll carry out those activities.

This will make it much simpler to get started right away and prevent one from putting things off.

5. Be willing to try new things: If you want to broaden your horizons, don't be afraid to branch out and participate in new kinds of activities or take up new kinds of interests.

This may assist you in finding new hobbies and passions that you can pursue when your dopamine detoxification is over.

Dopamine detoxification requires you to discover healthy alternatives, so keep this in mind as you go through the process.

You may achieve a better balance in your life and cut down on excessive stimulation if you replace activities that are too stimulating with ones that are healthier for you.

Practice self-care

Throughout the dopamine detox process, it is very necessary for both your physical and emotional health that you engage in self-care practices.

Throughout your time in detox, here are some measures that will assist you in practicing self-care:

1. Make getting enough rest and sleep a priority. Both your physical and mental health will benefit from getting an adequate amount of rest and sleep.

Establishing a consistent bedtime, cultivating an atmosphere conducive to restful sleep, and avoiding mentally taxing activities in the hours leading up to sleep should be your top priorities.

2. Participate in activities that promote relaxation Participating in activities that promote relaxation, such as yoga, meditation, and deep breathing, may assist you in lowering your levels of tension and anxiety while you are detoxing.

Include time in your calendar for these activities, and be sure to engage in them on a consistent basis.

3. Make sure you stay hydrated. In addition to being beneficial for your general health, drinking a lot of water will help you feel more energetic and focused while you are going through the detox process.

Drink at least eight full glasses of water every single day.

4. Consume a food that is balanced Consuming a diet that is balanced and consists of lots of fruits, vegetables, and whole grains helps provide your body with the nutrients it needs to perform at its best.

Avoid meals that have been processed, as well as sugar and caffeine, since they may all contribute to feeling overstimulated.

5. Get regular physical activity: Frequent exercise will help you decrease stress and anxiety, improve your mood, and raise your energy levels. If you want to enhance your mood and boost your energy levels, you should get regular exercise.

Choose a kind of physical exercise that you take pleasure in doing, such as walking, running, or dancing, and set some time in your week for it.

6. Make connections with other people Making connections with other people throughout your detox might offer you with emotional support and help you remain motivated.

Set up time on your calendar to hang out with friends or family, or sign up for a support group to meet other people who are also going through the dopamine detox process.

Do not forget that engaging in activities that promote your own well-being is an essential component of your dopamine withdrawal.

You may lessen feelings of stress and worry, increase the amount of energy you have, and create a better overall balance in your life if you take care of both your physical and mental health.

CHAPTER SIX

Assess your progress

Assessing how far you've come while going through dopamine withdrawal is a key part in the process of ensuring that you are staying on track and making progress toward achieving your objectives.

The following are some methods that can assist you in evaluating how far you have come:

1. Maintain a diary: Keeping a journal throughout your detox will help you monitor your progress and provide you an opportunity to reflect on the experiences you have had during the process.

You should write down your objectives, difficulties, and achievements, and then utilize this data to assess your overall development.

2. Make use of a checklist: When you begin your detox, make a checklist of the behaviors or routines that you want to eliminate from your life and the healthy alternatives that you want to replace them with.

Mark off each item on the checklist as you finish it, and then use it to track your progress and see where you stand.

3. Keep an eye on your state of mind and pay attention to how much energy you have Pay attention to how you feel and how much energy you have when you are detoxing.

Do you have a greater sense of energy and concentration today?

Are you finding that you are less stressed and anxious these days?

Make an assessment of your development with the use of this data.

4. Ask for input: Ask for comments from those who are helping you throughout your detoxification process.

Inquire about their impressions of your performance, and use their responses to help you assess how far you've come.

5. Be willing to make necessary adjustments to your plan: If you discover that your present strategy is not working or that you are not making progress towards your objectives, be willing to make necessary adjustments to your plan.

Find the areas in which you need to make adjustments, and then devise a new strategy that will assist you in accomplishing your objectives.

Keep in mind that monitoring your advancement during the dopamine withdrawal process is an essential component of the treatment.

You can remain on track and make progress toward your objectives if you keep track of your progress, evaluate your mood and energy levels, and ask for feedback.

What may be anticipate

Dopamine detox carried out in the manner described above is likely one of the most effective strategies to reestablish a healthy connection with the digital world. This was discussed in the previous section.

Be aware that the first few days may be challenging, and prepare yourself accordingly.

You will suffer from boredom.

To their good fortune, the vast majority of patients get relief rather quickly.

In a few of days, you'll find that even the most mundane tasks start to seem more enjoyable again.

Later on, you will feel less stressed out, have a greater feeling of control over the situation, and develop more patience.

Your ability to focus for longer periods of time will improve with time.

Some individuals first feel energized and full of passion for what they are doing, but after a few days this feeling fades and the task at hand becomes more challenging for them.

Prepare yourself for the possibility that it may be challenging for some time before it becomes easier.

Always tell yourself that the effort will be well worth it in the end.

After going through it yourself, you will be able to comprehend its meaning.

Imagine how wonderful it would be when seemingly little things, like going on a stroll in the woods, enjoying a meal, or listening to music, will make you happy.

Consider how satisfying it would be to keep the commitments you've made to do the chores that you said you would.

Imagine how good it would feel when you won't have to rush away to be distracted but instead will be able to sit quietly with your thoughts since you won't have to do that anymore.

CHAPTER SEVEN

Conclusions and helpful hints

In conclusion, dopamine detox is an effective method that may assist you in lowering your stress levels, enhancing your concentration, and developing a more healthy sense of equilibrium in your life.

The following are some concluding considerations and suggestions that will assist you in getting the most out of your dopamine detox:

1. Practice patience and don't give up: Dopamine detox is not a fast cure, and it may take some time before you start seeing the effects you desire.

Maintain patience and tenacity, and steadfast dedication to the accomplishment of your objectives.

2. Be aware of the things that set off your reactions:

Find out what behaviors, routines, or settings set off your dopamine response, and try to stay as far away from them as you can while you are detoxing.

3. Look for healthy alternatives: Instead of depending on activities or routines that produce dopamine, look for healthy alternatives that might deliver comparable advantages.

This might include activities such as going for a run, meditating, or spending time outside.

4. Engage in self-care activities Throughout the dopamine detox process, engaging in self-care activities is critical to both your

physical and emotional well-being.

Make getting enough rest and sleep a top priority, as well as maintaining a healthy diet and engaging in consistent physical exercise.

5. Maintain your connections: Speak with individuals who are through dopamine detoxification at the same time as you, or look for support from your friends and family.

Having a network of people who have your back might help keep you motivated and accountable.

Dopamine detox is a process, so keep in mind that it might take some time and work before you get the benefits you're looking for.

Focus on the good alterations that are taking place in your life, while also practicing patience, persistence, and kindness toward yourself.

You may realize your ambitions and create a life that is both healthier and more well-balanced with commitment and perseverance.

Summary

You don't feel good about how you spend your time, you aren't even enjoying it, and you behave compulsively on a regular basis; these are all symptoms that you may require a dopamine detox. The signs of an addiction are quite similar.

Dopamine detox may be a catchphrase, but the approach is based on cognitive behavior therapy, which is very successful for treating addiction of any kind, including internet addiction.

Dopamine detox is a short-term remedy that might assist you in reevaluating your connection to various electronic gadgets.

Try it out as a scientific experiment.

Examine the ways in which you spend your time when you are not forced to scroll constantly.

About The Author

Castro Atkin is a health and wellness expert with a passion for helping others achieve their goals and live their best lives. With over 10 years of experience in the health and wellness industry, Castro has developed a deep understanding of the connection between physical and mental well-being.

As a certified health coach and personal trainer, Castro has helped countless clients overcome stress, anxiety, and other challenges to achieve their goals and create a healthier, more balanced lifestyle. He is also a prolific writer and speaker, with a mission to share his knowledge and expertise with others.

In his latest book, "Dopamine Detox Guide," Castro shares his insights and expertise on one of the most powerful tools for reducing stress, improving focus, and creating a healthier balance in your life. With practical tips and step-by-step guidance, this book is the ultimate guide to dopamine detox, and a must-read for anyone looking to take control of their life and achieve their goals.

The End

9 798890 020017

Printed by Libri Plureos GmbH in Hamburg,
Germany